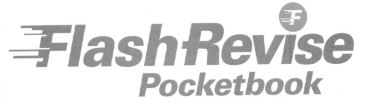

GCSE Phys
Education

G000066521

Philip Allan Updates, an imprint of Hodder Education, an Hachette UK company, Market Place, Deddington, Oxfordshire OX15 0SE

Orders

Bookpoint Ltd, 130 Milton Park, Abingdon, Oxfordshire OX14 4SB
tel: 01235 827827   fax: 01235 400401   e-mail: education@bookpoint.co.uk

Lines are open 9.00 a.m.–5.00 p.m., Monday to Saturday, with a 24-hour message answering service. You can also order through our website: www.philipallan.co.uk

© Philip Allan Updates 2009
ISBN 978-1-4441-0182-9

First published in 2006 as *Flashrevise Cards*

Impression number   5 4 3 2
Year   2015

Printed in India

Hachette UK's policy is to use papers that are natural, renewable and recyclable products and made from wood grown in sustainable forests. The logging and manufacturing processes are expected to conform to the environmental regulations of the country of origin.

P02024

Benefits of healthy, active lifestyles

Q1 Explain the meaning of a 'healthy, active lifestyle'.

Q2 The benefits of taking part in sport or physical activity can be classified under three different headings. Name each heading.

Q3 There is one more reason for taking part which is associated with appreciation of performance. What is it?

ANSWERS

A1 A lifestyle that contributes positively to physical, social and mental wellbeing. It includes regular exercise and physical activity

A2 Physical, social, mental (psychological)

A3 Aesthetic appreciation (or aesthetic)

***examiner's* note** People take part in sport and physical activity for physical, social and mental reasons and because they appreciate the beauty of the performance. You may be asked questions about the 'reasons for' or the 'benefits of' of taking part.

Reasons to participate in sport and physical activity

Q1 Give two physical reasons for taking part in sport and physical activity.

Q2 Give two social reasons for taking part in sport and physical activity.

Q3 Give two psychological (mental) reasons for taking part in sport and physical activity.

Q4 What is meant by aesthetic appreciation?

ANSWERS

A1 Choose from: to feel good; to improve fitness; to improve performance; physical challenge; contribution to good health; to improve a health-related exercise factor

A2 Choose from: to make friends; social mixing; membership of club or society; cooperation; working with others

A3 Choose from: relieves stress/anxiety; enjoyment; psychological challenge; competition; increases self-esteem

A4 Appreciating the beauty of the performance

***examiner's* note** People take part in sport for physical, social and psychological reasons and for aesthetic appreciation. The reasons for taking part and the benefits gained are very similar.

 ANSWERS

Psychological, physical and social benefits

Q1 Which of the following describes a psychological (mental) benefit of exercise: making new friends, enjoyment, improving fitness or physical challenge?

Q2 Which of the following describes a physical benefit of exercise: making new friends, enjoyment, improving fitness or cooperation?

Q3 Which of the following describes a social benefit of exercise: making new friends, enjoyment, improving fitness or improving flexibility?

Q4 Would 'relieving stress' be a social, psychological or physical benefit?

ANSWERS ▶▶

A1 Enjoyment

A2 Improving fitness

A3 Making new friends

A4 Psychological

examiner's **note** The benefits of exercise can be given as reasons for participation in sport and physical activity. Similarly, the reasons for participation include the benefits of exercise.

Influences on participants in physical activity I

There are six key areas of influence on those who take part in sport and physical activity.

Q1 Name three influences that come under the 'people' title.

Q2 Name two influences that come under the 'image' title.

Q3 Name four influences that come under the 'cultural' title.

ANSWERS

A1 Family, peers, role models

A2 Fashion, media coverage

A3 Age, disability, gender and race

***examiner's* note** These are recall questions, usually worth 1 mark each, but these often lead on to further marks. For example, questions may have a second part that requires you to add an explanation of your answer to the first part. A second part like this is usually worth more than 1 mark. Similar answers may also be acceptable, e.g. 'friends' in A1 above.

Influences on participants in physical activity II

Q1 Name four influences that come under the 'resources' title.

Q2 Name two influences that come under the 'health and well-being' title.

Q3 Name two influences that come under the 'socio-economic' title.

ANSWERS

A1 Access, availability, location, time

A2 Illness and health problems

A3 Cost and status

examiner's **note** These are recall questions, usually worth 1 mark each, but these often lead on to further marks. For example, questions may have a second part that requires you to add an explanation of your answer to the first part. A second part like this is usually worth more than 1 mark. Similar answers may also be acceptable.

Influences: family, peers and role models

Q1 Explain how family can influence you taking part in sport.

Q2 Explain how peers can influence you taking part in sport.

Q3 Explain how role models can influence you taking part in sport.

ANSWERS ▶▶

A1 Tennis star Andrew Murray was influenced by his mother, who was a coach. She took him to the tennis club and taught him to play at a very young age

A2 If your friends like a sport, you may want to go along and be with them. They may persuade and encourage you to take part

A3 Role models are often portrayed in the media. Seeing them performing excellently, winning competitions and being paid well may make you want to do the same and have the same fame and lifestyle

***examiner's* note** To answer these questions, there may be famous examples you can talk about, or you can explain from your own experience.

Roles in sport

Q1 Taking part in sport does not only mean being a performer. Name three other roles that you could play.

Q2 What qualities do you need to be a good leader?

Q3 What qualities do you need to be a good official?

Q4 What qualities do you need to be a good volunteer?

ANSWERS

A1 Leader, official or volunteer

A2 You must know the sport, have experience of playing it at some level and be good at motivating people

A3 You must know the rules and be firm, honest and consistent in making decisions

A4 You must be good with people, like the sport and know about it, and want to help others

examiner's **note** There may be other answers similar to the ones given that will get marks.

7 **ANSWERS**

The sports participation pyramid

The sports participation pyramid has four levels, as illustrated in the diagram. Name each one, starting with the lowest.

Q1 4?

Q2 3?

Q3 2?

Q4 1?

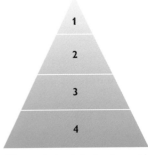

The sports participation pyramid

ANSWERS ▶▶

A1 Foundation

A2 Participation

A3 Performance

A4 Elite

examiner's **note** You should know the pyramid and the terms, and be able to explain them.

Levels of the pyramid

Q1 Explain what is meant by the foundation level.

Q2 Explain what is meant by the participation level.

Q3 Explain what is meant by the performance level.

Q4 Explain what is meant by the elite level.

ANSWERS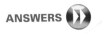

A1 This level is the base of the pyramid, where there are lots of participants learning and experiencing basic sporting skills

A2 This is the stage when people begin to participate regularly in a specific activity for enjoyment purposes

A3 During this stage, participants start to concentrate on specific sports and skills

A4 This is the peak of the pyramid, where individuals achieve sporting excellence

examiner's **note** The answers may not be exactly in these terms but should mean the same things.

 ANSWERS

PESSCL

Q1 What do the initials PESSCL stand for?

Q2 The main aim of the PESSCL programme is to get young people into sport in any of four roles. Name the four roles.

Q3 Another aim of the programme is to link sport in schools to what other area of participation?

ANSWERS

A1 Physical Education School Sport and Club Links

A2 Performers, leaders, officials and volunteers

A3 Club sport or club-level participation

***examiner's* note** You should know the initiative by its full title, not just the initials, as well as understand its aims.

Start, stay, succeed

Sport England has an initiative called 'start, stay, succeed'.

Q1 Explain what it means by START.

Q2 Explain what it means by STAY.

Q3 Explain what it means by SUCCEED.

ANSWERS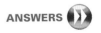

A1 Increase participation in sport to improve the health of the nation

A2 Retain people in sport through networks of clubs and facilities, coaches, volunteers and competitive opportunities

A3 Provide star performers with opportunities to succeed

***examiner's* note** The answers do not have to be in these exact words, but they should mean the same as the ones given.

 ANSWERS

Health, exercise, fitness and performance

Q1 Define the term 'health'.

Q2 What is exercise?

Q3 What do we mean by fitness?

Q4 What is performance?

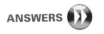
ANSWERS

A1 A state of complete physical, social and psychological (mental) wellbeing; not simply the absence of disease and infirmity

A2 A form of physical activity performed primarily to improve health and fitness

A3 The ability to meet or cope with the demands of the environment

A4 How well a task is completed

***examiner's* note** Health, exercise, fitness and performance are basic elements of sport. Exercise improves your health and fitness and will help you to perform better. Both the definition of health and the reasons for participation in sport include social and psychological elements as well as physical factors.

Health-related exercise I

There are five health-related
exercises:

1 CV

2 MS

3 ME

4 FL

5 BC

Q1 What does each of the
abbreviations stand for?

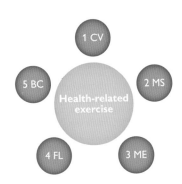

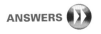

A1 1 Cardiovascular fitness

   2 Muscular strength

   3 Muscular endurance

   4 Flexibility

   5 Body composition

examiner's **note** This is a graphic organiser and a good way to remember the terms in the examination.

Health-related exercise II

Q1 How many health-related exercise factors are there: five, six, seven or eight?

Q2 Define cardiovascular fitness.

Q3 Define muscular strength.

Q4 Define muscular endurance.

ANSWERS ▶▶

A1 Five

A2 The ability to exercise the whole body for long periods of time

A3 The ability of the muscles to exert force against a resistance

A4 The ability of the voluntary muscles to work for long periods without getting tired

***examiner's* note** Health-related exercise is important in our daily lives and affects our performance in sport and physical activity. If you know how many health-related fitness factors there are, it will help you to remember them in the examination.

Health-related exercise III

There are five health-related exercise factors, including **cardiovascular** fitness, muscular strength and muscular endurance.

Q1 Which of the other two health-related exercise factors is more likely to be improved through yoga?

Q2 Define the health-related exercise factor from Question 1.

Q3 Identify the remaining health-related exercise factor.

Q4 Define the term identified in Question 3.

ANSWERS

A1 Flexibility

A2 The range of movement about a joint

A3 Body composition

A4 The percentages of fat, muscle and bone in the body

***examiner's* note** Flexibility and body composition are the most forgotten health-related exercise factors but they are important and complement the other three elements.

Health-related exercise IV

Q1 Name three activities that will improve cardiovascular fitness.

Q2 Name three activities that will improve muscular strength and muscular endurance.

Q3 Name three activities that will improve flexibility.

Q4 Name three activities that will improve body composition.

ANSWERS

A1 Choose from: swimming; cycling; running; jogging; walking; aerobics

A2 Choose from: weight training; multigym; circuit training; gymnastics; body pump

A3 Choose from: yoga; stretching; pilates; gymnastics

A4 Exercise; diet; energy balance (diet and exercise); weight training

***examiner's* note** It is important to be able to associate each activity with the particular area of health-related exercise that it is designed to improve. Some activities will improve more than one area. For example, gymnastics will improve muscular strength and endurance, as well as flexibility.

Health-related exercise V

Q1 Give two examples of health-related fitness factors that these players would need in order to improve their performance. Look for the most obvious.

Q2 Explain your answers to question 1.

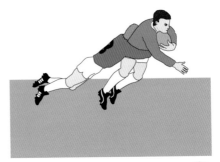

ANSWERS

A1 Cardiovascular fitness and muscular endurance

A2 Cardiovascular fitness would enable the players to keep running for the duration of the game; muscular endurance would enable them to compete strongly in the types of situation that arise throughout the game

examiner's **note** An explanation of your chosen answer may be required in an exam. Try to use the most obvious answer, as it is normally the easiest to explain.

Health-related exercise VI

Q1 Give two examples of health-related fitness factors that would be important for a gymnast.

Q2 Explain your answers to question 1.

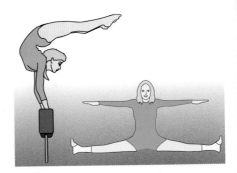

ANSWERS

A1 Muscular strength and flexibility

A2 Muscular strength is needed to hold difficult positions, such as a handstand, while flexibility is required to bend and stretch the body in order to get into positions such as the splits

examiner's **note** It is important to match the training to the requirements of the sport, e.g. muscular strength to gymnastics.

Skill-related fitness 1

Skill in sport is vital, and there are six main skill-related exercise terms. (Note that it is important not to mix these up with the health-related exercise terms.)

Q1 List the six skills in alphabetical order.

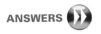
ANSWERS

A1 1 Agility

2 Balance

3 Coordination

4 Power

5 Reaction time

6 Speed

***examiner's* note** Only these six are acceptable as skill-related fitness terms. If you use any others or get them mixed up with the health-related terms, the answer will be marked as wrong.

Skill-related fitness II

Q1 How many skill-related exercise factors are there: five, six, seven or eight?

Q2 Define agility.

Q3 What is meant by reaction time?

Q4 Which skill-related fitness factor can be described as: 'the ability to perform strength movements quickly'?

ANSWERS

A1 Six

A2 The ability to move and change a body position quickly and in a controlled way

A3 The time between the presentation of a stimulus and the start of movement

A4 Power

examiner's **note** Questions on health-related and skill-related factors in sport are almost always included in the exam and examiners point out that many candidates get confused between the two. It is therefore important to know which terms are health-related and which are skill-related. It may help if you remember that there are five health-related factors and six skill-related factors.

Skill-related fitness III

Q1 Define speed.

Q2 Which skill refers to the ability to use two or more body parts together?

Q3 Which skill refers to the ability to retain the body's centre of gravity above the base of support (while still or moving)?

Q4 Define power.

ANSWERS ▸▸

A1 The rate at which an individual is able to perform a movement or cover a distance

A2 Coordination

A3 Balance

A4 Strength × speed

examiner's **note** Some of these definitions are quite difficult to learn and you are not usually required to give them in the examination. However, you should be able to recognise them.

Skill-related fitness IV

Q1 Name a sport that requires agility. Explain your answer.

Q2 Name a sport that requires coordination. Explain your answer.

Q3 Name a sport that requires a quick reaction time. Explain your answer.

Q4 Name a sport that requires power. Explain your answer.

ANSWERS

A1 Football — a player moves his whole body, at speed and under control, in order to dodge past an opponent

A2 Cricket — a fielder sees the ball come off the bat and follows it with his eyes in order to catch it with his hands

A3 Sprinting (100 m) — the sprinter hears the stimulus (the gun) and starts to run immediately

A4 Rugby — a player runs with the ball and, as he is tackled, continues to drive over the line for a try

examiner's **note** When you are asked to choose a sport, don't just state the name of the sport, e.g. football — show how the skill is used in that activity, e.g. (for speed) sprinting past a defender into space to get the ball.

Applying skill-related fitness 1

Q1 Which skill is the most useful for a gymnast doing a handstand on the beam?

Q2 Which skill is the most useful for a table-tennis player returning a fast smash by her opponent?

Q3 Which skill is the most useful for a weightlifter lifting a heavy weight?

Q4 Which skill is the most useful for a cricketer trying to stop the ball reaching the boundary?

ANSWERS

A1 Balance

A2 Reaction time or coordination

A3 Power

A4 Speed

***examiner's* note** It is important to go for the most obvious answer as this will be the easiest to apply to the move or stroke that the performer is making. Choosing a less obvious skill is much more difficult to justify and is not what the examiner is looking for. However, there may be more than one obvious answer, as in Question 2.

Applying skill-related fitness II

Four skill-related factors are given below. Match each of these factors to the most appropriate sport listed in Questions 1–4.

power   agility   speed   coordination

Q1 .... is most useful for trampolining.

Q2 .... is most useful for shot put.

Q3 .... is most useful for tennis.

Q4 .... is most useful for long jump.

ANSWERS ▶▶

A1 Agility

A2 Power

A3 Coordination

A4 Speed

examiner's **note** Although in this instance the skills are actually given, the same points apply as in Topic 23 — go for the most obvious answer. You must make sure that all the skills can be applied to the appropriate sport — if you get one wrong, it will affect your answers to the other questions.

Applying skill-related fitness III

Four sports are given below. Match each of these sports to the most appropriate skill-related factor listed in Questions 1–4.

netball   golf   sprint swimming   high jump

Q1 .... most relies on reaction time.

Q2 .... most relies on power.

Q3 .... most relies on balance.

Q4 .... most relies on coordination.

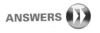
ANSWERS

A1 Sprint swimming

A2 High jump

A3 Golf

A4 Netball

***examiner's* note** When matching skill-related fitness factors to different sports, it is important to use your knowledge and experience of your own specialist games and activities — team games such as netball, individual sports such as golf and popular activities such as swimming and athletics. If you do not have specialist knowledge of these games or activities, you will be able to apply your knowledge as long as you understand the skills.

It will help you if you put the obvious answers in first (e.g. power = high jump), especially if you are not familiar with one of the sports.

Applying skill-related fitness IV

Q1 Speed aids performance in sprinting. It helps by getting the runner to the finish line quickly. Name a sport in which agility helps performance.

Q2 Explain how agility helps the performer.

Q3 Name a sport in which balance helps performance.

Q4 Explain how balance helps the performer.

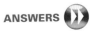

ANSWERS ❯❯

A1 Gymnastics

A2 It helps by controlling the whole body when performing moves in a floor routine

A3 Gymnastics

A4 It helps to hold a handstand on the beam or when landing from a move

***examiner's* note** When asked to match the skill to the sport and then *explain* how it is used, model your answer on the example given. Go for the most obvious sport, which will probably be the easiest to explain.

Explaining skill-related fitness I

Q1 Name a sport in which reaction time helps performance.

Q2 Explain how reaction time helps the performer.

Q3 Name a sport in which power helps performance.

Q4 Explain how power helps the performer.

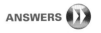

ANSWERS

A1 Football

A2 It helps the goalkeeper save penalties by moving as soon as the ball is struck

A3 Hammer throwing

A4 The hammer thrower rotates quickly around the circle and pulls on the hammer with great strength — power = strength × speed

***examiner's* note** These questions are similar to those in Topic 26 but with different skills, so again, choose an obvious sport which will be the easiest to *explain*.

Explaining skill-related fitness II

Q1 Explain how speed helps the performer in rounders.

Q2 Explain how coordination helps the performer in rounders.

Q3 Explain how speed helps the performer in tennis.

Q4 Explain how coordination helps the performer in tennis.

ANSWERS ▶▶

A1 It helps the player reach the base quickly or to run fast in order to score a rounder after hitting the ball

A2 It helps the player watch the ball onto the bat in order to hit it as far as possible

A3 It helps the player get into position quickly in order to return a shot

A4 It helps the player watch the ball onto the racket in order to return a shot

examiner's **note** These specific questions are designed to stretch you in order to achieve higher marks. Such questions do not allow you to choose your own sport, so they are more difficult.

Understanding skill-related fitness

Q1 Which skill-related fitness factor is essential to a sprinter when the gun fires and he starts to move?

Q2 Which skill-related fitness factor is defined by strength × speed?

Q3 Which skill-related fitness factor is the ability to move two or more body parts together?

Q4 Which skill-related fitness factor is essential in sport when you are still or on the move?

ANSWERS

A1 Reaction time

A2 Power

A3 Coordination

A4 Balance

examiner's **note** In this type of question there is only one acceptable answer, whereas in the earlier questions on skill-related fitness there is often more than one correct response. It is therefore important to understand each of the six skill-related factors.

Applying knowledge from each section

Q1 Sarah is a gymnast and has to perform at a high level. Although the competition is hard, she feels that she gets some psychological (mental) benefits from it. Name two of these possible benefits.

Q2 What term is used to describe an appreciation of the beauty of Sarah's performance?

Q3 Explain how exercise and fitness combine to improve her performance.

Q4 Sarah needs power when she performs the vault, but at what precise moment does she use this?

ANSWERS

A1 Choose from: relief of stress/anxiety; enjoyment; psychological challenge; competition

A2 Aesthetic appreciation

A3 When Sarah exercises, it improves her fitness and this enables her to meet the demands of the activity better

A4 As she hits the board at take-off

***examiner's* note** This question combines several topics built into a scenario, and you may find similar ones in the examination. Although the sport mentioned may not be one which you specialise in, you should be able to apply the knowledge you have gained from the theory parts of the course to the question.

Preparing to perform a personal exercise programme

Q1 What do the letters PARQ stand for?

Q2 Why is it important for a person to complete a PARQ form before starting a personal exercise programme?

Q3 All PARQ forms contain a question on which major body organ?

Q4 What test would a doctor use to assess the fitness of this organ?

ANSWERS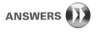

A1 Physical Activity Readiness Questionnaire

A2 To make sure that there is no reason why he or she should not take part in exercise or physical activity

A3 The heart

A4 Taking the person's blood pressure

examiner's note You may devise your own PARQ, but there is a basic format that they should all conform to. Sample PARQs can be found on the internet and you could use them to check your answers.

Fitness testing for health-related exercise 1

Five tests used to check fitness levels for health-related exercise are:
1 grip strength test; 2 sit and reach test; 3 Harvard step test; 4 body mass index (BMI); 5 maximum press-ups in 30 seconds.

Q1 Which test would you use for cardiovascular fitness?

Q2 Which test would you use for muscular strength?

Q3 Which test would you use for muscular endurance?

Q4 Which test would you use for flexibility?

Q5 Which test would you use for body composition?

ANSWERS))

A1 Harvard step test

A2 Grip strength test

A3 Maximum press-ups in 30 seconds

A4 Sit and reach test

A5 Body mass index

examiner's **note** These are standard tests that you may perform as a practical activity.

Fitness testing for health-related exercise II

Q1 How many minutes does the Cooper's run test last for?

Q2 What factor of health-related exercise is it testing?

Q3 How can taking a test before starting a personal exercise programme help to motivate you?

Q4 Briefly explain the Cooper's run test protocol, i.e. how to do it.

ANSWERS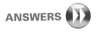

A1 **12**

A2 Cardiovascular fitness

A3 It gives you a baseline level of fitness which you can aim to improve by the end of the programme

A4 You run on a set course for 12 minutes, then measure and record how far you have run

examiner's **note** You should know the tests and how to perform them, as well as how they may be used in a personal exercise programme. This may be how they are tested in the examination.

Fitness testing for skill-related fitness 1

Which of the following skills is being checked by the test in each question?

agility, balance, coordination, power, reaction time, speed

Q1 Standing broad jump?

Q2 Sergeant jump?

Q3 Three-ball juggle?

Q4 Stork stand?

ANSWERS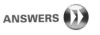

A1 Power

A2 Power

A3 Coordination

A4 Balance

***examiner's* note** As stated earlier, you must know the six skill-related fitness factors. Here, you need to be able to match them to the correct tests.

Fitness testing for skill-related fitness II

Q1 Suggest a suitable test for each of the skills listed below.

agility   reaction time   speed

Q2 Explain briefly how the sergeant jump test is performed.

ANSWERS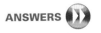

A1 Illinois agility run; ruler drop test; 30 m sprint

A2 Put some chalk dust on your finger tips, then stand next to a wall, reach as high as possible and touch the wall (or the sergeant jump board, set at 0 where you reach). Then jump as high as possible and touch the wall or board. Make sure some chalk rubs off and measure the distance between your standing mark and jumping mark. This is your sergeant jump score

***examiner's* note** This question tests the remaining skills and is more difficult as the tests are not given, so you must know what they are.

Principles of training I

Q1 How many principles of training are there — five, six, seven or eight?

Q2 The first principle that people often apply to their training programme is the one that makes it applicable to them personally. What is this principle called?

Q3 What does FITT stand for?

Q4 By doing a personal exercise programme to improve in a particular sport or activity, which principle of training are you applying?

ANSWERS

A1 Seven

A2 Individual needs

A3 Frequency, intensity, time, type

A4 Specificity

examiner's **note** You need to know how many principles of training there are, what each one is and how to apply them — e.g. how they would be used to plan a personal exercise programme.

Principles of training II

The principles of training are as follows: recovery; rest; reversibility; FITT; individual needs; progressive overload; specificity.

Q1 Which principle should you apply in order to keep getting gradually fitter?

Q2 When starting a training programme, which principle should you apply to make sure your body gets time to repair any damage caused and for adaptations to take place?

Q3 If you train too hard or get injured, which principle of training might take effect?

Q4 Which principle refers to the period of time allotted to recovery?

ANSWERS

A1 Progression overload

A2 Recovery

A3 Reversibility

A4 Rest

examiner's **note** You may also have used the principles of training when performing your personal exercise programme, so you should get all these questions right.

Principles of training III

Q1 Which principle of training should be used to allow the body to repair damage caused by training or competition?

Q2 Jack is a sprinter and in his training he concentrates on improving his speed. What principle of training is he applying?

Q3 Explain how you could tell from Jack's personal exercise programme that he was applying the principle of progressive overload.

Q4 Give an example of how you could see that he was using this principle of training.

ANSWERS

A1 Recovery

A2 Specificity

A3 His programme would show that his training was gradually getting harder

A4 He could train more often (frequency) and/or train at a higher intensity, e.g. he could run faster

***examiner's* note** You have probably not done methods of training yet, but should be able to apply your knowledge of the FITT principle here.

Principles of training IV

John has been training for and competing in the triathlon — running, swimming and cycling. Now, he wants to focus on his cycling.

Q1 John trained using a swimming pool, treadmill, exercise bicycle and rowing machine. Which should he concentrate on now?

Q2 Which principle of training is being applied?

Q3 Explain why he should concentrate his training in this way.

Q4 After 4 weeks, John notes that his fitness has improved. What principle must he use to take his fitness to the next stage?

ANSWERS

A1 Exercise bicycle

A2 Specificity

A3 By using this machine, he is training in a way that most resembles the activity he will be competing in

A4 Progressive overload

***examiner's* note** When a question is asked about activities with which you are not familiar, e.g. the triathlon, simply use your knowledge and apply it to the situation. It is important to know how progressive overload is used.

Principles of training V

John, a triathlete, wants to develop his training programme to improve his fitness further. To do this, he could apply the FITT principle of training.

Q1 How can frequency be used to develop his fitness?

Q2 How can intensity be used to develop his fitness?

Q3 How can time be used to develop his fitness?

Q4 How can type be used to develop his fitness?

ANSWERS

A1 He could train more often, e.g. more times each week

A2 He could train harder or faster, e.g. by cycling up hills

A3 He could train for longer periods of time, e.g. 25 minutes instead of 20

A4 He could use interval training as the type of training he is doing

***examiner's* note** FITT is a four-part principle and may be set as a whole question or as individual parts. Type is linked to the methods of training and your ability to use your knowledge of that area of the specification as well using the principles of training.

Principles of training VI

Q1 Which principle of training must you apply to make sure you continue to improve your fitness?

Q2 Which principle applies if you stop training?

Q3 Which principle describes the process of repairing any damage caused when undertaking a personal exercise programme?

Q4 Which principle describes the period of time needed to allow Q3 to take place?

ANSWERS

A1 Progressive overload

A2 Reversibility

A3 Recovery

A4 Rest

examiner's **note** Q1, Q3 and Q4 are new principles of training in the specification, so you need to learn these and know how they are applied.

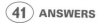

Goal setting: SMART goals

Goal setting is performed using the acronym SMART.
What does each letter stand for?

Q1 S

Q2 M

Q3 A

Q4 R

Q5 T

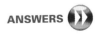
ANSWERS

A1 Specific

A2 Measurable

A3 Achievable

A4 Realistic

A5 Time-bound

examiner's **note** You should use goal setting during your course, e.g. when developing your personal exercise programme.

Goal setting for your personal exercise programme

What do the following terms mean when setting goals for a personal exercise programme:

Q1 Measurable?

Q2 Achievable?

Q3 Realistic?

Q4 Time-bound?

ANSWERS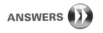

A1 It should be possible to perform a test at the start of the programme and then re-test in the same way (using the correct protocol) at the end of the programme to measure whether a goal has been achieved

A2 Goals should not be so difficult that it is impossible for you to reach them by the end of your programme

A3 Goals set should be actually within your grasp, not just wishful thinking

A4 If a programme is set to last a period of 6 weeks, that is how long you have to achieve your goals

***examiner's* note** It is important both to know what each letter stands for in the acronym and to be able to explain how they can be used, e.g. how you used them in your personal exercise programme.

Methods of training

Q1 Explain what is meant by circuit training.

Q2 What type of training is generally done at a constant, steady pace, with no rest periods?

Q3 What is Fartlek training?

Q4 What type of training involves periods of high-intensity work followed by short rest periods?

ANSWERS

A1 A series of exercises designed to exercise the whole body in such a way that each muscle group is rested after it has been worked

A2 Continuous training

A3 Training using changes of speed, e.g. run fast, run slow, run fast, walk, jog, usually performed over varying terrains (e.g. through woods, up hills)

A4 Interval training

examiner's **note** Each training method has specific characteristics. The particular method of training chosen by an athlete depends on the required outcome.

Matching methods to activities

Match each training method with the most obvious sport. Use each method only once.

interval; continuous; Fartlek; circuit training

Q1 Swimming

Q2 Sprinting

Q3 Badminton

Q4 Marathon running

ANSWERS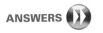

A1 Circuit training

A2 Interval

A3 Fartlek

A4 Continuous

examiner's **note** This is the type of question that you might get in the examination, and you need to go for the most obvious first, e.g. matching sprinting to interval training, then marathon running to continuous training. That leaves badminton and swimming, Fartlek and circuit training. Swimming fits best with circuit training, therefore leaving badminton with Fartlek.

Applying methods of training

Q1 Which of the following are methods of training: specificity; interval; health-related exercise; Fartlek; continuous; FITT?

Q2 Which method of training involves 'speedplay'?

Q3 Which method of training involves using heavy weights and few repetitions?

Q4 What is the term for a combination of two or more training methods?

ANSWERS

A1 Interval; Fartlek; continuous
A2 Fartlek training
A3 Weight training
A4 Cross training

***examiner's* note** It is important that you show some understanding of the different methods of training. You should be able to describe and explain specific activities and consider the advantages and disadvantages of each method.

Circuit training

Q1 In circuit training, what is the name given to each location where an exercise takes place?

Q2 Give an example of an exercise for the arm muscles.

Q3 Give an example of an exercise for the leg muscles.

Q4 Give an example of an exercise for the abdominal muscles.

ANSWERS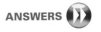

A1 Station

A2 Press-ups

A3 Step-ups

A4 Sit-ups

examiner's **note** In circuit training, the athlete performs a series of exercises in a particular order. Each exercise concentrates on a different muscle group to allow for recovery. Questions 1–4 are examples of the easier type of exam question which do not test your knowledge of muscles and muscle groups. In the harder questions, you will have to apply your knowledge of anatomy, physiology and circuit training.

Circuit training: applying your knowledge I

Q1 Why is it important in circuit training to exercise different muscle groups in successive exercises?

Q2 Give an example of an exercise to improve the fitness of the heart.

Q3 When performing a press-up, which two muscles in the arms work together in pairs to bend and straighten the arm?

Q4 When performing a squat, which two muscles in the legs work together in pairs to bend and straighten the leg?

A1 To allow the different muscle groups to rest and recover

A2 Shuttle runs

A3 Biceps and triceps

A4 Quadriceps and hamstrings

examiner's **note** Circuit training exercises should include arm, leg, trunk and cardiovascular exercises. Questions 1–4 are examples of the harder type of exam question. Here, you are expected to apply your knowledge of muscles and appropriate exercises for them.

Circuit training: applying your knowledge II

Q1 When performing a press-up, what name is given to the type of muscle contraction that occurs when movement takes place?

Q2 When a press-up is held in a static position for a few seconds with the arms straight, what type of muscle contraction occurs?

Q3 Give an example of an adapted exercise (made easier) for a person who cannot perform the exercise as it would normally be performed.

Q4 Give an example of an adapted exercise (made more difficult) for a person who finds the exercise too easy.

ANSWERS

A1 Isotonic

A2 Isometric

A3 Adapted press-up — a press-up in a kneeling position

A4 Adapted press-up — a press-up with feet on a bench and hands on the floor

examiner's **note** The resistance used in press-ups, squats etc. is the athlete's body weight. Questions 1–4 are examples of the harder type of exam question. These questions test your knowledge of anatomy, physiology and circuit training, and your ability to adapt exercises for both weaker and stronger performers.

Interval training

Q1 What is the name given to one performance of a task, e.g. a 300 m run?

Q2 What is the name given to groups of, say, four such tasks, separated by periods of rest?

Q3 Which athlete would be more likely to use interval training to improve his performance: a marathon runner or a 400 m runner?

Q4 In an interval training session, what happens to the athlete's heart rate during the recovery period?

ANSWERS

A1 **A repetition**

A2 **Sets**

A3 **400 m runner**

A4 **Slows down**

***examiner's* note** Interval training is when a training session is divided into a series of repetitions and sets. It is used to improve the performer's speed. Questions on repetitions and sets can be applied to a variety of training methods, for example the number of times a press-up is performed in circuit training. In weight training, it could refer to a bench press or, for a swimmer, the number of lengths or distance.

Analysing an interval training session

Sarah completed an interval training session using a heart rate monitor. Her results are shown in the graph.

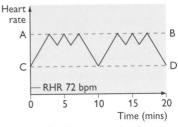

Sarah's training chart

Q1 How many repetitions has Sarah completed altogether? Explain your answer.

Q2 How many sets did she perform? Explain your answer.

Q3 The title under the graph indicates that Sarah is using a particular principle of training. Which one is it?

 ANSWERS

A1 Six repetitions. There are six peaks when her heart rate was high, showing that she was working at a very high intensity

A2 Two sets. After the third high-intensity repetition, she has a low heart rate and a longer rest period, indicating that she had a break between the two sets

A3 Individual needs

examiner's **note** You need to be able to understand graphical information such as that used to monitor various training methods. Once again, a question has appeared requiring knowledge from another part of the course, this time from the principles of training.

More methods of training

Q1 A person swims at a constant pace for 20 minutes. What type of training is this?

Q2 Apart from swimming, give two other activities that use this training method.

Q3 Which athlete would be more likely to use this training method to improve her performance: a marathon runner or a 400 m runner?

Q4 Which aspect of health and fitness would be most improved by this type of training?

ANSWERS

A1 Continuous

A2 Choose from: jogging, walking, cycling, rowing or similar

A3 Marathon runner

A4 Cardiovascular fitness

examiner's **note** Continuous training involves exercise without rest intervals. It is mostly used to improve aerobic fitness. The principles of training must be applied in order to gain improvement in aerobic fitness.

Weight (resistance) training: applying your knowledge I

Q1 Weight training can be used to improve which two obvious factors of health-related exercise?

Q2 From the diagram, explain which two muscles are working, 1 to stand in the upright position and 2 to lower into the squat position.

Q3 Name the term used to describe muscles working in this way.

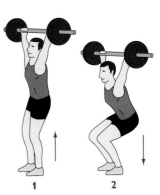

1   2

ANSWERS

A1 Muscular strength and muscular endurance

A2 1 quadriceps, 2 hamstrings

A3 Antagonistic

***examiner's* note** These are similar questions to those that are likely to come up in questions on circuit training, requiring you to apply knowledge in the same way.

Weight (resistance) training: applying your knowledge II

Q1 Which muscle is used to hold the weight in position 1 and in position 2?

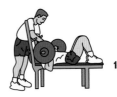

1

Q2 Name the term used to mean working the bar up and down without stopping.

Q3 Name the term used to mean holding the bar still at the top of the movement.

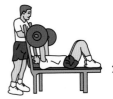

2

ANSWERS ▶▶

A1 **1 Biceps, 2 triceps**

A2 Isotonic

A3 Isometric

examiner's **note** If you learn the muscles and use the terminology in this part of the course, you will find it easier to answer the questions in the examination.

Methods of training: applying your knowledge

The five athletes listed below are training for the Olympic Games. Choose a suitable training method for each. Use each training method only once.

fartlek, weight lifting, continuous, interval, circuit

Q1 100 m swimmer

Q2 1500 m runner

Q3 Hockey player

Q4 Weight lifter

Q5 Badminton player

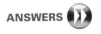

ANSWERS

A1 Interval training

A2 Continuous training

A3 Fartlek training or circuit training

A4 Weight lifting

A5 Circuit training or Fartlek training

examiner's **note** The weight lifter needs strength, so the most obvious method is weight lifting. Do that question first. then allocate the next obvious ones, e.g. the swimmer needs speed, so interval is the obvious method. The 1500 m runner also needs speed but continuous is the most obvious answer. Fartlek and circuit training will fit either the hockey or badminton players, but Fartlek is probably best to give to the hockey (games) player and circuit to badminton.

Applying your knowledge so far I

Q1 Explain how a circuit training session might result in a social benefit of exercise.

Q2 Explain how an interval training session might provide a mental benefit of exercise.

Q3 Explain how a continuous training session might bring about a physical benefit of exercise.

ANSWERS ▶▶

A1 Circuit training often takes place indoors with large numbers of people, so you would be working and cooperating with others

A2 Interval training is high intensity, which can produce the hormone serotonin – the feel-good hormone

A3 Continuous training helps to improve cardiovascular fitness

***examiner's* note** It is important that you know how methods of training can improve health and fitness by helping to develop physical, social and mental capacity.

Applying your knowledge so far II

Q1 Explain how circuit training can be used to improve two different aspects of your health-related fitness.

Q2 Name two exercises that can be used to improve two different aspects of your skill-related fitness.

Q3 Choose a sport and explain a skill practice that you could include in a circuit-training session for that sport.

Q4 Name and explain a skill practice that you could include in a circuit-training session for a different sport.

ANSWERS

A1 Circuit training improves cardiovascular fitness over a period of time, keeping your heart rate in the target zone. Muscular endurance is also improved by exercises, e.g. bench dips

A2 Choose from: agility – the agility ladder; balance – the tree position in yoga; coordination – three-ball juggle; power – burpees; speed – shuttle runs

A3 Basketball – you could jump shots around the key then move on when you score from that position

A4 Hockey – you could incorporate dribbling around a line of cones using reverse stick

***examiner's* note** You need to be able to link methods of training to specific activities, based upon the requirements of health-related exercise and skill-related fitness.

Warming up and cooling down

Q1 Name the three parts of an exercise session.

Q2 Name the three parts of a warm-up, in the correct order.

Q3 Give three reasons why you should warm up.

Q4 Give one reason for a cool down.

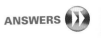
ANSWERS

A1 Warm-up, main activity and cool down

A2 Pulse-raising activity, stretching and then skills related to the activity, e.g. sprinter practising a sprint start

A3 Choose from: it raises the heart rate; prevents injury; prepares you psychologically, results in better performance

A4 Choose from: disperses lactic acid; brings the heart rate gradually back to resting rate

examiner's **note** You must know how to plan an exercise session and the purpose of each component: warm-up, main activity and cool down.

Using the principles of training in a personal exercise programme 1

Q1 Louise is following a 6-week personal exercise programme that her coach has devised for her. Which principle of training is she using?

Q2 In the first 2 weeks, she works at 60%–70% of her target zone. In the next 2 weeks, she works at a higher range.
(a) What principle of training is she using?
(b) Which part of the FITT principle is she applying?

Q3 In the last 2 weeks she trains with her heart rate in the target zone for 25 minutes instead of 20 minutes. Which part of the FITT principle is she using now?

ANSWERS

A1 Individual needs

A2 (a) Progressive overload (b) I – intensity

A3 T – time

***examiner's* note** You need to know how to explain the use of the principles of training in an exercise programme and how these can improve health-related fitness. List the principles and work through them to make sure you choose the correct one to answer the question. It will help to have a set pattern of how to work through the principles, so you do not miss one out.

Using the principles of training in a personal exercise programme II

Q1 Louise is going to use continuous training as part of her programme. What part of the FITT principle is she applying?

Q2 Because as she is a 1500 m runner, this type of training suits what she needs for her event. What principle of training is she using?

Q3 So that she doesn't overdo things, Louise's coach wants her to have a day off between each training session to allow her body to repair the damage caused by hard training. What principle of training are they applying now?

Q4 What principle is used to allow this period of time where damage is repaired?

ANSWERS

A1 T – type

A2 Specificity

A3 Recovery

A4 Rest

***examiner's* note** You need to know how to explain the use of the principles of training in an exercise programme and how these can improve fitness. List the principles and work through them to make sure you choose the correct one to answer the question. It will help to have a set pattern of how to work through the principles, so you do not miss one out..

Analysing the FITT principle

Q1 Using the FITT principle, is John working at a high, low or medium intensity during this session?

Q2 Explain your answer.

Q3 Using the T for time in the FITT principle, how long was John's heart rate in the required area?

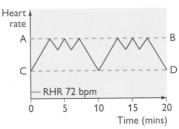

John's training chart

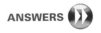

A1 High intensity

A2 AB represents the 80% training threshold line and John's heart rate reaches this line six times during the training period, so he is working very hard

A3 20 minutes

examiner's note To get high marks, you may be required to explain some simple graphical data. You should also be able to do simple calculations, using the data in the graph.

Aerobic and anaerobic activity

weight training; interval training; Fartlek training;
continuous training; circuit training

Q1 Which of the above training methods is the most obvious to use to improve anaerobic fitness?

Q2 Explain your answer.

Q3 Which of the above training methods is the most obvious to use to improve aerobic fitness?

Q4 Explain your answer.

ANSWERS

A1 Interval training

A2 Interval training is short, fast bursts of high-intensity exercise, which means the performer will be breathless and short of oxygen (anaerobic means 'without oxygen')

A3 Continuous training

A4 Continuous training is performed at a steady rate and does not involve high-intensity work, so the performer does not become breathless. The exercise is done 'with oxygen', which is the meaning of aerobic

***examiner's* note** You must be able to link methods of training to aerobic and anaerobic activity.

Exercise and heart rate

The graph shows Louise's heart rate during a training session.

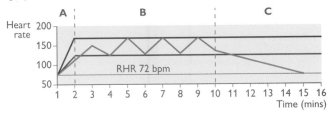

Q1 Name the terms used to describe her heart rate
(a) before she starts to exercise (b) during exercise
(c) when she stops exercising

ANSWERS

A1 (a) Resting heart rate
   (b) Working heart rate
   (c) Recovery rate

***examiner's* note** You must understand what is meant by resting heart rate, working heart rate and recovery rate, and be able to plot examples on a graph and evaluate results.

Graphical analysis I

The graph shows Louise's heart rate during a training session.

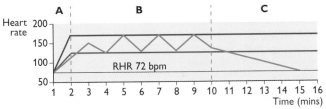

Q1 Name the parts of the training session A, B and C.

Q2 What was Louise's highest heart rate? When was this reached?

Q3 How long did it take for her heart rate to return to normal?

ANSWERS

A1 Warm up, main activity and cool down
A2 **167 bpm** (must have 'bpm' or not correct, just writing '167' is not good enough); in the ninth minute
A3 **6 minutes**

examiner's note You must be able to recognise the parts of a training session: warm up, main activity and cool down.

Graphical analysis II

Q1 What is the area between the lines AB and CD called?

Q2 This training chart is for Anita, aged 16. How are the positions of the lines AB and CD calculated?

Q3 How do we know that Anita is working at a worthwhile intensity?

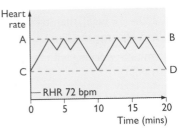

Anita's training chart

ANSWERS ▶▶

A1 The target zone

A2 220 – 16 (age); then take 80% of this calculation for the line AB and 60% for the line CD

A3 Anita is working with her heart rate between the thresholds of training.

***examiner's* note** It is unlikely that you will have to calculate the target zone for a performer of a given age in the exam, but you should know the formula.

Graphical analysis III

Q1 What is the name given to the lines AB and CD?

Q2 What importance do they have in a training session?

Q3 What two parts of the FITT principle is Anita using during her training session?

Q4 Explain your answer.

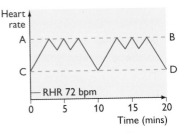

Anita's training chart

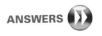

A1 Thresholds of training

A2 As a minimum, Anita's heart rate should be between these two lines during her training session

A3 Intensity and time (could also be type, as she is using interval training)

A4 Intensity: we can see that Anita's heart rate is going up very high, so she is working at a high intensity

Time: she has worked for 20 minutes with her heart rate in the target zone. (If type is given, then it is because she is using interval training)

***examiner's* note** In a question like this, go through the four parts of the FITT principle to see which are being used., starting with the F for frequency. That is not being used here, so go on to the next letter and so on.

Graphical analysis IV

Q1 What training method is Anita using?

Q2 Explain your answer.

Q3 How many repetitions and sets has she done?

Q4 Explain your answer.

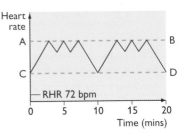

Anita's training chart

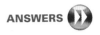

ANSWERS ⟩⟩

A1 Interval training

A2 She is working at a high intensity, then resting and allowing her heart rate to come down, then working at a high intensity again. This is the definition of interval training

A3 Six repetitions and two sets

A4 She has six peaks where she has worked really hard, with a period between the first and second sets of three peaks when her heart rate has come down further, showing she has had a longer rest between two sets

examiner's **note** You need to be able to analyse a lot of information from the charts across the specification, to show a deeper understanding and an ability to apply your knowledge.

Graphical analysis V

Q1 Which method of training is Anita most likely to be using if her heart rate measurements produce the graph shown?

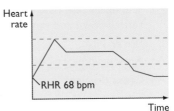

Q2 Explain your answer.

Q3 This graph has been drawn after 6 weeks of training. Explain why Anita's resting heart rate is lower than it was in Topic 65.

Q4 Anita has now used more than one method of training. What is this type of training called?

ANSWERS

A1 Continuous training

A2 The heart rate rises quickly at the start of training and then settles down and remains constant as the athlete works at a steady pace

A3 A reduced heart rate indicates improved fitness levels

A4 Cross training

examiner's **note** The two most common graphs used in this type of question are for interval training and continuous training. However, other training methods may also be used, so you should be familiar with the shapes that all types of training graphs produce.

Graphical analysis VI

Q1 Anita does exactly the same training session 2 weeks later, but this time her recovery rate is quicker.
What does this indicate?

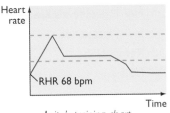

Anita's training chart

Q2 The title under the graph indicates that Anita is using which principle of training?

Q3 If she were to train too hard and get injured, which principle is likely to take effect?

Q4 Which principle of training could Anita use to allow her body time to recovery from her training?

ANSWERS

A1 Her fitness levels are improving

A2 Individual needs

A3 Reversibility

A4 Rest

examiner's **note** On occasion, you will be given a scenario and required to use your knowledge to answer several different questions about it.

Factors of a balanced diet

Q1 What are the three macro nutrients of a balanced diet?

Q2 Which food group would you associate with a Sumo wrestler, a sprinter or strong man and a marathon runner?

Q3 Which other nutrient would be important to a marathon runner before and during a race, and why?

Q4 Describe the conditions that might make this nutrient even more important.

ANSWERS

A1 Carbohydrates, protein and fat

A2 Sumo wrestler: fat; sprinter or strong man: protein;
marathon runner: carbohydrate

A3 Water, to prevent dehydration

A4 Heat and humidity

***examiner's* note** You need to know that there are seven factors of a
balanced diet and that they a split into smaller groups, such as macro and micro
plus water and fibre. You should also know which food groups are associated
with specific sports, such as protein and muscle building, and understand the link
between exercise, diet, work and rest.

Diet, sport and physical activity

Q1 Name two food groups, other than carbohydrates, that an athlete can use as a source of energy.

Q2 Name the two micro nutrients.

Q3 Give an example of a food that is rich in carbohydrate.

Q4 Explain why is it important to eat 2–3 hours before taking part in sport and physical activity.

ANSWERS

A1 Fat and protein

A2 Vitamins and minerals

A3 Bread, rice, potatoes, pasta

A4 Food should be taken at least 2 hours before taking part in sport and physical activity because when you start to exercise, blood is sent to the muscles (blood shunting) and less is available to digest food. This may cause cramps and discomfort

***examiner's* note** You should know the food groups and the importance of each in sport and physical activity, as well as understand the need to eat at the appropriate time before exercise and why.

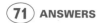

The effect of diet on health

Q1 Which mineral is closely linked to keeping our bones healthy?

Q2 Which vitamin combines with this mineral for strong bones and teeth?

Q3 Give an example of a food that is rich in vitamins.

Q4 Give an example of a food that is rich in protein.

Q5 Explain what might happen if a person does not keep to a good energy balance in respect of their diet and exercise.

ANSWERS

A1 Calcium

A2 Vitamin D

A3 Fruit, vegetables

A4 Meat, fish, dairy products, nuts, cereals

A5 If someone takes in more calories than they use, they put weight on. If they burn up more calories than they take in, they will lose weight

examiner's **note** For Q3 and Q4, you may give other acceptable answers or specific answers, e.g. oranges for Q3.

Body types

The term somatotype is used to describe a person's body type.

Q1 Which somatotype describes a thin body?

Q2 Which somatotype describes a fat body?

Q3 Which somatotype describes a muscular body?

Q4 Which somatotype is a jockey most likely to have?

ANSWERS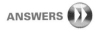

A1 Ectomorph

A2 Endomorph

A3 Mesomorph

A4 Ectomorph

***examiner's* note** You need to understand what is meant by the term 'somatotype' and be able to describe the different body types, referring to the extreme forms — endomorph, mesomorph and ectomorph. Most people are not an extreme form but a combination of types. For example, a person may be an endomorphic mesomorph, meaning that his/her main score is in mesomorphy (or muscle) with some endomorphy (fat).

Somatotypes and their sports

Q1 Which somatotype is likely to make the best high jumper?

Q2 Explain your answer.

Q3 Which somatotype is likely to make the best sprinter?

Q4 Explain your answer.

ANSWERS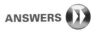

A1 Ectomorph

A2 They are likely to be tall and slim with less weight to raise over the bar

A3 Mesomorph

A4 They will be well muscled, strong and powerful and not carrying too much extra weight

***examiner's* note** The sport a person takes part in, or in some cases the position he/she plays, is often related to somatotype. You need to be aware of which sport or position the various somatotypes are generally most suited for and the reasons for this.

The somatochart

Q1 Which somatotypes appear at positions A, B and C?

Q2 Where on the somatochart would a muscular boxer be placed?

Q3 Where on the somatochart would a tall, slim basketball player be placed?

Q4 Where on the somatochart would a sumo wrestler be placed?

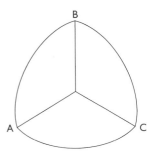

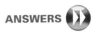

ANSWERS

A1 A — endomorph; B — mesomorph; C — ectomorph

A2 Position B

A3 Position C

A4 Position A

***examiner's* note** A somatochart is used for displaying body types. You should
know where on the somatochart each of the extreme body types —
endomorph, mesomorph and ectomorph — can be found. Most people fall in
the areas between the extremes.

Body weight and sport

Q1 Explain why two people of the same height may be different weights but both may still be a suitable weight for their height.

Q2 Explain how this might affect the sports that people play.

Q3 What is the name for the eating disorder that is due to loss of appetite?

Q4 Explain what is meant by the term 'optimum weight'.

ANSWERS

A1 They may be of different sexes or have a different bone structure and muscle girth

A2 Some sports need people to be heavier than others, e.g. rugby forwards are strong and powerful but are heavier than most people of their height

A3 Anorexia (nervosa)

A4 The weight most suited to enabling you to give your best performance in your sport

***examiner's* note** You will need to know that height, gender, bone structure and muscle girth can affect your weight. People vary and you must be able to explain the implications of this.

Overweight, overfat, obese

Q1 Explain the term 'overweight'.

Q2 Explain the term 'overfat'.

Q3 Explain the term 'obese'.

Q4 Explain which of these conditions is the most harmful and why.

ANSWERS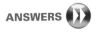

A1 A person who weighs more than normal for his or her height, but who does not have too much body fat; not harmful if not too much of the weight is fat

A2 A person who has more body fat than he or she should have for their height and weight, but not excessive

A3 A person who is very overfat (or grossly overfat), having much more of their weight as fat than they should have

A4 Obesity is the most harmful because it puts extra stress on the body and the organs, especially the heart

***examiner's* note** Overweight does not necessarily mean that a person has too much body weight as fat. A well-built person, toned with well-developed muscles, may be heavier because muscle weighs more than fat.

Socially acceptable drugs

Q1 Drugs can fall into two categories: those that are socially acceptable and those that are socially unacceptable. Name a drug that is considered to be socially acceptable.

Q2 For the drug you have named in Question 1, give a possible side effect.

Q3 Name another drug that is considered to be socially acceptable.

Q4 For the drug you have named in Question 3, give a possible side effect.

ANSWERS

A1 Alcohol

A2 Liver or kidney disease; high blood pressure

A3 Nicotine

A4 Heart disease; high blood pressure; lung cancer; damaged alveoli

***examiner's* note** Socially acceptable drugs also include caffeine (found in tea, coffee and cola drinks) and drugs prescribed for colds and flu. Smoking is sometimes given as an answer when a drug is asked for, but smoking is not a drug — nicotine is the required answer. You may be asked questions on the effects that nicotine and alcohol have on performance in sport and physical activity, as well as the effects they have on general health.

Performance-enhancing drugs

Q1 Give one reason why athletes take illegal performance-enhancing drugs.

Q2 Anabolic steroids are drugs that some athletes take to improve their performance. What effect do these drugs have on the athletes' training potential?

Q3 Give an example of an event in which athletes might take steroids to improve their performance.

Q4 EPO is a type of drug. Give an example of an event in which athletes might take this drug.

ANSWERS

A1 To win, or to be able to compete at the top level
A2 The athletes can train harder for longer and recover more quickly
A3 Any strength event, or sprinting — but not long-distance events
A4 Distance events in which cardiovascular endurance is important, such as long-distance cycling races

***examiner's* note** Certain drugs that are considered to be performance enhancing are illegal and are on what is known as the 'banned list'. Some of these are dangerous and some are not. However, some top athletes and games players still use these drugs and risk being banned from their sport.

Drugs and health

Q1 Why might athletes use an analgesic?

Q2 Give an example of a harmful side effect of taking this type of drug.

Q3 Why might an athlete use a diuretic?

Q4 Give an example of a harmful side effect of taking this type of drug.

ANSWERS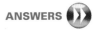

A1 To relieve or mask a painful injury, so that they can still perform

A2 An athlete may compete and make the injury worse

A3 To lose weight

A4 Dehydration

***examiner's* note** You are more likely to be asked questions on the general categories of drugs, such as stimulants, analgesics, anabolic steroids and diuretics, rather than on a specific drug such as nandrolone. EPO (erythropoietin) may be the exception to this.

Prevention of sports injuries

Q1 Choose a sport and explain how its rules can help to prevent injury.

Q2 For the sport chosen in Question 1, give two items of clothing that help to prevent injury.

Q3 For the sport chosen in Question 1, give two competition rules that help prevent injury during a match or game.

Q4 Give another two further competition rules that are designed to prevent injury to the participants (these may come from sports other than the one chosen in Question 1).

ANSWERS

A1 Football; if players commit a foul (which may result in injury to the opponent), a free kick is awarded against them, which may result in a goal. For a serious offence, players may also be booked or even sent off. This may deter them from fouling again.

A2 Football boots and shin pads

A3 For football matches: same-sex games, i.e. boys play boys, girls play girls; players of a similar age compete against each other

A4 Grading, e.g. judo; weight categories, e.g. boxing

***examiner's* note** Be careful which sport you choose when answering this type of question — some sports are easier to apply the answers to than others. The rules of the game are there not just to decide who has won but also to help prevent injury.

A healthy, active lifestyle and your cardiovascular system

Q1 Name three components of the cardiovascular system.

Q2 Give three immediate effects of exercise.

Q3 Blood pressure is a measure of the fitness of the heart.
Give the names of the two components of blood pressure.

Q4 What effect is alcohol consumption likely to have on a person's blood pressure?

Q5 What immediate and long-term effects will exercise and physical activity have on your blood pressure?

ANSWERS

A1 The heart, the blood and the blood vessels

A2 The heart beats faster and more strongly, and blood pressure may rise

A3 Systolic and diastolic

A4 It will cause it to go up

A5 During exercise it will go up, but over long term it will gradually come down

examiner's **note** Cardiovascular fitness is an important aspect of health-related exercise, so you should know the components of the cardiovascular system as well as the immediate effects of exercise and the effects it can have on blood pressure in the long term.

Exercise and your cardiovascular system

Q1 Give three long-term benefits of exercise to the cardiovascular system.

Q2 What name is given to the volume of blood pumped with each heart beat?

Q3 What name is given to the volume of blood pumped by the heart each minute? How is this increased during exercise?

Q4 What is the formula that links heart rate with the two previous answers?

ANSWERS

A1 Any three from: increased stroke volume; increased cardiac output; decrease in resting heart rate; faster recovery rate; cardiac hypertrophy; reduced risk of CHD; lower blood pressure; improved ability to transport oxygen; healthy veins and arteries

A2 Stroke volume

A3 Cardiac output; it increases as the heart beats faster

A4 heart rate × stroke volume = cardiac output

examiner's **note** The number of times the heart beats per minute (heart rate), the volume it pumps per beat (stroke volume) and the volume it pumps per minute (cardiac output) are related. You need to understand exactly how the three terms are linked (by the formula); how one affects the other, and how they are used in a practical context in sport, physical activity and training.

Cholesterol, arteries and the respiratory system

Cholesterol in our diet can be good or bad for our arteries. One type is thought to be good cholesterol and the other is thought to be bad.

Q1 What is the good cholesterol called?

Q2 What is the bad cholesterol called?

Q3 Give three immediate effects of exercise on the respiratory system.

Q4 Give three long-term benefits of regular exercise on the respiratory system.

ANSWERS

A1 High density lipoprotein (HDL)

A2 Low density lipoprotein (LDL)

A3 Choose from: increased breathing rate; increased breathing depth; oxygen debt

A4 Choose from: more efficient lungs; stronger diaphragm/intercostal muscle; increased tidal volume; increased vital capacity; more efficient gaseous exchange; increased capilliarisation of alveoli; creation of more alveoli

examiner's **note** HDL and LDL would be sufficient to get a mark in most cases. You need to know both the immediate and long-term effects of exercise, including specific terms.

Exercise and your respiratory system

Q1 What name is given to the amount of air inspired and expired with each normal breath?

Q2 What name is given to the largest amount of air that can be made to pass into and out of the lungs by the most forceful inspiration and expiration?

Q3 Explain what is meant by the term 'oxygen debt'.

Q4 Who would be more likely to experience oxygen debt — a sprinter or a marathon runner?

ANSWERS

A1 Tidal volume

A2 Vital capacity

A3 More oxygen is consumed during recovery than would be consumed in the same length of time at rest. This results in a shortfall of oxygen available

A4 Sprinter

examiner's **note** Tidal volume and vital capacity are terms linked to the respiratory system. They are also linked to exercise and training in that they increase as fitness improves.

Your cardiovascular and respiratory systems

Q1 Name the term that is being defined by each of the following:

A – amount of oxygen consumed during recovery above that which would have ordinarily been consumed in the same time at rest

B – amount of air inhaled and exhaled with each normal breath

C – with oxygen

D – volume of blood pumped with each beat of the heart

E – largest amount of air that can be made to pass into and out of the lungs by the most forceful inhalation and exhalation

F – without oxygen

G – volume of blood pumped by the heart each minute

ANSWERS

A1 A oxygen debt
    B tidal volume
    C aerobic
    D stroke volume
    E vital capacity
    F anaerobic
    G cardiac output

***examiner's* note** There are always multiple-choice questions on the exam paper and these are some of the terms that come up in this context.

Types of muscle

Q1 There are three different types of muscle, which have different functions. Explain what skeletal muscles are.

Q2 What other name are they known by?

Q3 What name is given to the muscle type over which we have no control?

Q4 What name is given to the third type of muscle? Explain how it is different from the other two types.

ANSWERS

A1 They are attached to the skeleton and we can control their actions

A2 Voluntary

A3 Involuntary

A4 Cardiac/heart muscle. It is not under our conscious control but it continues to work as long as it has a good blood supply

examiner's **note** You need to know how muscles are linked to other areas of the specification: how muscles can be trained to improve muscular strength and endurance; and how flexibility can be improved. You also need to know about different muscle actions. Muscles and drugs are linked too in terms of training and the use of anabolic steroids.

Muscle fibres

Q1 Name the two types of fibre in skeletal/voluntary muscles.

Q2 Take one of these and give an example of an athletic event in which you would expect the competitors to have more of this type of fibre.

Q3 Give an example of an athletic event in which you would expect the competitors to have more of the other type of fibre.

Q4 Explain what is meant by an isotonic muscle contraction.

ANSWERS

A1 Fast twitch and slow twitch

A2 Fast twitch — 100 m (any short, fast event)

A3 Slow twitch — 5000 m (any slow, long-distance event)

A4 When a muscle is contracted and a movement takes place,
     e.g. kicking a football

***examiner's* note** The ratio of the two different types of fibre that make up muscles can influence the sports that we are good at. You need to be able to apply this knowledge to particular sporting activities.

Muscles of the body I

Q1 Name the three muscles A, B and C.

Q2 What must a muscle do for movement to take place?

Q3 Which of these muscles is responsible for raising your arm above your head?

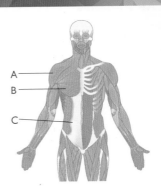

A

B

C

ANSWERS ▶▶

A1 A = deltoid
    B = pectorals
    C = abdominals

A2 Contract

A3 A — deltoid

examiner's **note** You are required to know these muscles of the body. You must know the names of the muscles, where in the body they are and which muscles are responsible for specific actions or movements. Students often forget the importance of the term 'muscle contraction' and the fact that muscles must contract for movement to take place.

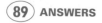

Muscles of the body II

Q1 Name the three muscles A, B and C.

Q2 Which of these muscles is exercised doing pull-downs on a weights machine?

Q3 Which muscle is responsible for lifting the leg straight backwards?

Q4 Complete this sentence:
For movement to take place, a muscle must ....

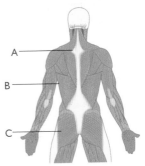

ANSWERS

A1 A = trapezius
    B = latissimus dorsi
    C = gluteus maximus

A2 B — latissimus dorsi

A3 C — gluteus maximus

A4 Contract

examiner's **note** Muscles are attached to bones by tendons. When a muscle contracts, it pulls on the bone it is attached to — so it can pull but it cannot push. No movement can take place without muscle contraction, and you need to know which muscle is responsible for a particular action.

Muscles of the arms

Q1 Name the muscles A and B.

Q2 Which of these muscles flexes the arm at the elbow?

Q3 Which of these muscles extends the arm at the elbow?

Q4 Explain the term antagonistic muscles and give an example of muscles that work in this way.

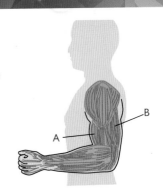

ANSWERS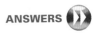

A1 A = biceps
    B = triceps

A2 A — biceps

A3 B — triceps

A4 Antagonistic describes the action of muscles working in pairs to produce opposite effects. Examples are the biceps and triceps or the quadriceps and hamstrings.

***examiner's* note** Throwing events, racket sports and fitness and training activities involve a great deal of action from the biceps and triceps, which cause actions such as flexion and extension at the elbow joint. In training activities such as weight training, they can be strengthened using specific exercises such as the biceps curl.

Muscles of the lower body and legs

Q1 Name the muscles A, B, C and D.

Q2 Which muscle is responsible for straightening the knee when kicking a football?

Q3 Which muscle is responsible for bending the knee when sprinting?

Q4 Which muscle is responsible for driving forward off the toes when running a marathon, for example?

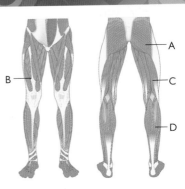

ANSWERS

A1 A = gluteus maximus
    B = quadriceps
    C = hamstring
    D = gastrocnemius

A2 B — quadriceps

A3 C — hamstring

A4 D — gastrocnemius

examiner's **note** The gluteals and leg muscles are responsible for the actions of running and jumping in many sports and physical activities such as rugby and netball, as well as individual sports such as sprinting and jumping events. Weight training exercises, such as step-ups and squats, can strengthen the leg muscles. Like the biceps and triceps, the quadriceps and hamstrings work together as an antagonistic pair.

Muscles: applying your knowledge

Q1 When performing press-ups, which muscle contracts as each arm straightens?

Q2 When muscles increase in size through exercise, what term is used to describe this effect?

Q3 What term is used to describe the reduction in muscle size due to lack of exercise?

Q4 Give two ways in which athletes would benefit from taking performance-enhancing drugs

ANSWERS

A1 Triceps

A2 Muscle hypertrophy

A3 Muscle atrophy

A4 They would be able to train harder/longer and recover more quickly, as well as developing bigger muscles

examiner's **note** You will not have to know the specific names of drugs, but you must know the types of drug that athletes use and their effects on performance and training. You should be familiar with the terms muscle hypertrophy and muscle atrophy.

Bones: long-term benefits of exercise

Q1 What is the condition that can affect our bones in old age?

Q2 What type of exercise can help prevent this condition?

Q3 Which type of exercise is best for bone health: swimming, treadmill, exercise bike or rowing?

Q4 Give three functions of the skeleton.

ANSWERS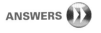

A1 Osteoporosis

A2 Weight-bearing exercise

A3 Treadmill

A4 Movement, support and protection

***examiner's* note** Age is a factor that affects performance and osteoporosis is a condition that can be improved with suitable exercise and diet.

Joints: long-term benefits of exercise

Q1 What is the definition of a joint?

Q2 What type of joint is found at the elbow and the knee?

Q3 What type of joint is found at the shoulder?

Q4 Give an example of the long-term benefits of exercise on bones.

Q5 Give an example of the long-term benefits of exercise on tendons.

 ANSWERS

A1 A place where two or more bones meet

A2 Hinge

A3 Ball and socket

A4 Increased bone density

A5 They become stronger

***examiner's* note** The three important joints that you must know are shoulder (ball and socket) and elbow and knee (hinge). You should know about the benefits of exercise for your bones, especially the importance of weight-bearing exercise.

Joint actions

Name the type(s) of joint action that occur in Questions 1–4.

Q1 At the knee when a footballer straightens her leg to strike the ball.

Q2 At the elbow when a table tennis player bends his arm at the elbow and then straightens it for a back-hand smash.

Q3 At the shoulder when a person doing astride jumps first takes her arms away from the body and then brings them back again.

Q4 At the shoulder when a bowler bowls a cricket ball.

ANSWERS

A1 Extension

A2 Flexion, extension — in this order

A3 Abduction, adduction — in this order

A4 Rotation

***examiner's* note** Joints allow a variety of movement and these questions test your knowledge of various sporting actions. When the angle at a joint gets bigger, the action is extension. When the angle gets smaller, the action is flexion. Joints are held together by ligaments, not tendons. Remember that flexibility is the amount of movement possible at a joint, and that flexibility at the joints is reduced by injury and age.

Sports injuries: signs and symptoms

Q1 If a player sustains an injury, there may be signs and/or symptoms. Explain the difference between a sign and a symptom.

Q2 There are four different types of fracture you need to know. Name one of them.

Q3 If a bone is only broken part of the way across, what kind of fracture is it?

Q4 Sometimes a severe blow can move a bone out of a joint. What is the term used to describe this type of injury?

ANSWERS

A1 A sign is what you can see, feel, hear or smell. A symptom is what the player will tell you about the injury

A2 Choose from: compound, stress, greenstick or simple

A3 Greenstick

A4 Dislocation

***examiner's* note** You need to know the different types of fracture, and it will help to know the signs and symptoms of each.

Types of sports injury

Q1 A strain and a sprain are not the same. Which is a possible joint injury?

Q2 If a tennis player has an elbow injury, what symptom will suggest to him that it is tennis elbow and where will this symptom occur?

Q3 If a golfer has an elbow injury, what symptom will suggest to her that it is golfer's elbow and where will this symptom occur?

Q4 Are tennis and golfer's elbow injuries to the ligaments, tendons or muscles?

ANSWERS

A1 Sprain

A2 Pain on the outside of the elbow

A3 Pain on the inside of the elbow

A4 Tendons

examiner's **note** Golfer's elbow and tennis elbow are examples of similar injuries but with different symptoms. Sprain and strain are often mixed up, but you must know which is which.

Treatment of sports injuries

Q1 The RICE principle is a term used to describe the treatment of some injuries. What does each letter stand for?

Q2 Give an example of an injury that this type of treatment would be used for.

Q3 What name is given to these types of tissue injury?

ANSWERS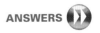

A1 Rest, ice, compression, elevation

A2 Choose from: sprains; strains; tennis or golfer's elbow

A3 Soft tissue injuries

***examiner's* note** RICE is the recognised treatment for soft tissue injuries. If the player receives an injury, he or she should stop playing (rest); ice should be applied to the injured area; a support bandage should be applied (compression) and the injured part should be elevated.

Tackling difficult
multiple-choice questions

For each question, read both statements and then decide whether:

A Both statements are correct.
B Statement (i) is correct and statement (ii) is incorrect.
C Statement (i) is incorrect and statement (ii) is correct.
D Both statements are incorrect.

	(i)	(ii)
Q1	Flexion means the angle at the joint gets bigger.	Extension means the angle at the joint gets smaller.
Q2	Adduction is when the limb is drawn towards the body.	Rotation is when the limb is moved in a circular motion.
Q3	Adduction is when the limb is taken away from the body.	Abduction is when the limb is taken away from the body.

ANSWERS

A1 D

A2 A

A3 C

examiner's **note** Students often find this type of multiple-choice question very difficult. You will find it much easier if you tick or cross each statement as you read it and then work out which of A, B, C or D is the right one.